A Shorter Course in

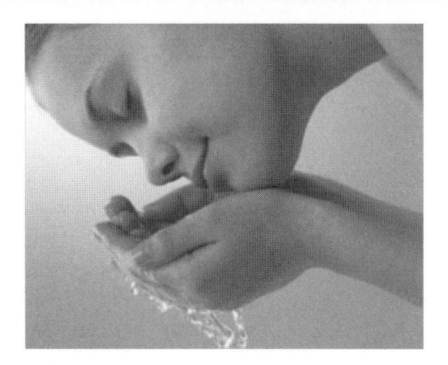

GOOD HEALTH

5分間　健康・医療・看護

Yukio Seya　Tsukimaro Nishimura　Jun Nakayama

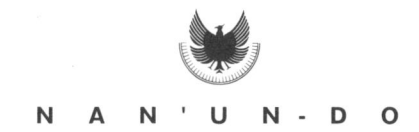

NAN'UN-DO

カセット・テープで予習，復習を。
《ヒアリングの力を飛躍的に伸ばすことができます》
本書には，自宅での予習復習用のカセット・テープが付属・別売されています。ぜひ，ご利用ください。（全1巻）
カセット・テープの収録箇所は，各 Chapter の
英文テキスト・他。

本書の構成と使い方

　本書は，主として我々現代人の心身の健康にまつわる up-to-date で一般的な問題を比較的平易な英語で論じた 42 の文章で構成され，更に，それに付随した応用問題とで編集しました。従って，医学，薬学，保健衛生学，看護学系の学生はもとより，文科系一般の学生諸君にとっても興味ある英語教材として利用できるものと思います。

　英語を習得するには，「読む」，「書く」，「聞く」，「話す」の 4 技能の運用能力を一様に養うことが大切なのは言うまでもありません。本書では特にこれらの点に留意して，できる限り総合教材としても利用できるよう工夫しました。

　先ず，Notes を参考にしてテキストを注意深く読み，内容を正確に理解するように努めてください。それを踏まえて，exercises では本文中の基本的な語句，イディオム，構文等を応用した数種の作文問題，ヒアリングの訓練を反復練習することによって，自分の意志を相手に直接伝える communication の能力を同時に培うよう心掛けてください。

　最後に，このテキストの上梓にあたり，惜しみない助言と協力をいただいた南雲堂学事部の橋本勇氏に心より感謝の意を表します。

編著者

CONTENTS

1. Smoking Danger　喫煙の危険 ……………………**6**
2. Healthy Vitamin C　ビタミンCと健康 ……………**7**
3. The Mystery of Vitamin C　ビタミンCの神秘 ………**8**
4. Safer Inhospital Environment　安全な病院内環境 ………**9**
5. Towards 2000 : the WHO Targets
   西暦2000年，WHOの目標 ……………………………**10**
6. Dental Hygienists　歯科衛生士の役割 ………………**11**
7. Amino Acids　未来の予防薬，アミノ酸 ………………**12**
8. The Pros and Cons of Abortion　人工中絶の賛否 ………**13**
9. The Effect of Laughter　笑いの効用 …………………**14**
10. How to Enjoy Drinking　酒の上手なのみ方 ……………**15**
11. How to Promote Health　健康増進のために ……………**16**
12. Vocational Rehabilitation Counselor
    社会復帰カウンセラー …………………………………**17**
13. Almighty Germanium　万能のゲルマニウム ……………**18**
14. Calcium and Adult Diseases　カルシュウムと成人病 ……**19**
15. Dr. Waksman, Father of Antibiotics
    抗生物質の父，ワクスマン博士 ………………………**20**
16. The Insulin Factory　インシュリン工場 ………………**21**
17. Unconscious Dying Patients　生命維持の是非 …………**22**
18. What Are Interferons?　インターフェロンとは ………**23**

19. Allergies　アレルギー体質 …………………………24
20. How to Lose Weight on a Diet　ダイエットによる減量 …25
21. The Mind-Body Effect　心と身体の関係 ………………26
22. Treatment of Child's High Fever　子供の高熱の手当……27
23. Mental Health　心の健康 ………………………………28
24. Prevention of Influenza　インフルエンザの予防 ………29
25. A War against AIDS　エイズとの戦い ………………30
26. Diet and Cancer　食事と癌 ……………………………31
27. The Nature of AIDS　エイズの性質 …………………32
28. German Measles　風疹 …………………………………33
29. What Should an A.I.D. Child Be Told?
　　精子提供者の匿名義務 …………………………………34
30. Factors of High Blood Pressure　高血圧の諸原因 ………35
31. A Godsend for Ulcers　潰瘍の天与の妙薬 ……………36
32. How to Thrive on Stress　ストレスを逆用する ………37
33. Heart Transplant　心臓移植 ……………………………38
34. Cell Division: Initiator of Life's Fire
　　生命の火を燃やすもの …………………………………39
35. The Black Death　黒死病 ………………………………40
36. Four Humors　4つの体液の意味 ………………………41
37. The Hospice Movement　ホスピス運動 ………………42
38. How We Get Old　老化の仕組 …………………………43
39. Plasticity in Brain Development　脳の発達 ……………44
40. How and Why Do We Dream?　夢の不思議 …………45
41. The Beveridge Plan　福祉国家をめざして ……………46
42. Liability of Nursing Staff　看護の意味 ………………47

1. Smoking Danger （喫煙の危険）

If you smoke—particularly cigarettes—you are far more likely than a non-smoker to suffer or die from several major diseases—notably lung cancer, coronary heart disease and chronic bronchitis. One smoker in four dies prematurely because of his smoking. The risk of dying for a heavy smoker (between the ages of 35 and 55) is roughly equal to the risk run by a non-smoker, 10 years older.

From another point of view: if you're 35 and smoke 25-plus a day, you have as much risk of dying before you're 44 as a Second World War serviceman had of being killed—about 1 in 22 in each case.

are likely to「～しそうである」 **far more than**「～より遙かに一層」 **notably** = especially. **die from**「～で死ぬ」 **coronary**「冠状動脈の」 **chronic bronchitis**「慢性気管支炎」 *cf*. acute「急性の」 **prematurely** = before the usual or proper time. **run**「(危険などを)冒す」 **From ～ point of view**「～の見地から見れば」

Exercise 1 : WRITING　（本文中の語句を参考にして、次の日本文を英文になおしなさい。）

1.　運動をし過ぎるとかえって身体を壊してしまうだろう。

2.　生命を危険にさらすような馬鹿なことはよせ。

3.　その作品は歴史的見地から極めて重要なものである。

2. Healthy Vitamin C （ビタミンCと健康）

To get an idea just how important vitamin C really is, imagine what would happen to your house if all the nails, glue, and cement were removed. The house would fall apart, of course. But imagine how bad the devastation would be if not only the nails, glue, and cement were removed, but the microscopic glue that holds the molecules of wood, mortar, and other materials was also removed. You'd be left with a pile of dust.

Vitamin C is essential to the formation of collagen, which is the fundamental glue of the body. Collagen is a protein that supports bone, skin, teeth, cartilage, tendon, and connective tissue. Without adequate vitamin C, the body begins literally to disintegrate into dust. Stress uses up vitamin C. Conversely, vitamin C supports our ability to withstand stress. Vitamin C also helps the cells breathe, and serves as a powerful antioxidant.

glue「接着剤」 **fall apart**「崩れおちる」 **microscopic**「極微の」 **molecules**「分子」 **a pile of**「～の山積み」 **collagen**「こう原質」 **cartilage**「軟骨」 **tendon**「けん」 *cf*. Achilles' tendon. **disintegrate**「分解する」 **antioxidant**「老化防止剤」

Exercise 2: LISTENING （テープを聞いて空所を埋め，和訳しなさい。）

1. When it comes to writing about vitamin C, we have no problem digging up (　　　) of the vitamin's usefulness to (　　　) good health.

2. Vitamin C boosts the immune system, encourages (　　　), supports (　　　), and helps us better withstand stresses of all kinds.

3. Vitamin C has shown (　　　) in prolonging the lives of (　　　) cancer patients, and it can lower insulin requirements for diabetics.

3. The Mystery of Vitamin C （ビタミンCの神秘）

　　Double Nobel Prize winner Linus Pauling is now advocating a new modern science of nutrition that would involve the use of large quantities of synthetic vitamins, especially C. He says, "Ascorbic acid, vitamin C is an extremely useful compound. There is some evidence that it helps in the prevention of cancer and there is very good evidence that it helps in the absorption of iron and vitamin A. When people get colds, they don't feel the symptoms as much with doses of vitamin C."

Linus Pauling (1901-) 米国の化学者。Nobel 化学賞(1954)，平和賞(1962)の両賞を受賞。 **advocate**「唱道する」 **nutrition**「栄養」 **synthetic**「合成した」 **ascorbic acid** = vitamin C 「アスコルビン酸」 **prevention**「予防」 **absorption**「吸収」

Exercise 3 : WRITING 　（与えられた書き出しを用いて，英訳しなさい。）

1. ビタミンEは皮膚の老化の予防に役立つという証拠がある。
   There is some evidence that...

2. ビタミンCをのむことにより人々はより健康になれると彼は結論を下している。
   With doses of vitamin C, he concludes, ...

3. 年度末試験がおわるまで風邪をひかないように気をつけなさい。
   Be careful not to ...

4. Safer Inhospital Environment （安全な病院内環境）

Though hospitals are supposed to be safe places where the injured or ill go to recover, the institutions may be filled with potential dangers for young patients. Possible hazards are dangerous radiators, unlocked medicine rooms, windows without screens, wet, slippery floors, sharp syringes or blades left out on patient tables.

These are due to either carelessness in normal day-to-day hospital routine or lack of understanding of the potential dangers to children within the hospital environment. Greater attention must be paid to keep hospitals safe for children.

the injured or ill「けが人や病人」 **hazard**＝danger. **potential**「潜在的な」 **syringe**「注射器」 **blade**「カミソリの刃」 **day-to-day hospital routine**「日々の病院の決まりきった仕事」

Exercise 4 : WRITING （日本語のヒントをもとに，英文を完成しなさい。）

1. Nurses ＿＿＿＿＿（3語）＿＿＿＿＿ be kind and considerate
   ［…なはずである］

   ＿＿＿＿＿（3語）＿＿＿＿＿
   ［自分達の患者に対して］

2. This accident is ＿＿＿＿＿（3語）＿＿＿＿＿ of all people involved
   ［不注意による］
   in this plan.

3. The classroom of pathology ＿＿＿＿＿（3語）＿＿＿＿＿ freshmen.
   ［一杯だった］

5. Towards 2000 : the WHO Targets (西暦2000年：WHOの目標)

In 1984 the European Region of the WHO drew up a strategy for attaining 'Health for All by the Year 2000' and in 1985 issued detailed targets to which the UK has agreed. Firstly, it acknowledged that there are certain fundamental conditions which have to be met before any real improvements can be made — the prerequisites for health :

* freedom from the fear of war ;
* equal opportunities for all ;
* satisfaction of the basic needs for food, basic education, clean water and sanitation, decent housing, secure work and a useful role in society ;
* political will and public support to launch the necessary action.

'Without peace and social justice, without enough food and water, without education and decent housing, and without providing each and all with a useful role in society and adequate income, there can be no health for the people, no real growth and no social development' (WHO 1985).

WHO＝World Health Organization「世界保健機関（1948年に設立）」 **draw up**「～を作成する」 **attain**「～を達成する」 **acknowledge**「～を認める」 **meet**「～に立ち向かう」 **prerequisites**「前提条件」 **sanitation**「公衆衛生」 **launch**「～を始める」 **decent**「きちんとした」 **adequate**「～に十分な」

Exercise 5 : WRITING (カッコ内の語(句)を用いて，英訳しなさい。)

1. 平和と正義がなければ社会の発展はありえない。(without)

2. "すべての人が健康に"がWHOの目標である。(target)

3. 人々は戦争の心配のない社会を望んでいる。(free)

6. Dental Hygienists （歯科衛生士の役割）

Chances are the person who cleans your teeth when you visit the dentist is not a dentist, but a dental hygienist. These auxiliary health professionals assist dentists in their practice by providing direct dental services, such as taking X-rays, cleaning teeth, applying fluoride or other materials to make the teeth resistant to decay, examining teeth, and performing various laboratory tests. In addition, hygienists educate patients about good oral health and the relationship between diet and oral health.

But the practice of dental hygiene is changing. In many states, hygienists now perform expanded functions that were formerly performed by the dentist alone, such as administering local anesthetics, placing dressings on wounds following surgery, and placing and removing temporary tooth restorations.

chances are「おそらく…だ」 **auxiliary**「補助の」 **practice**「業務」 **fluoride**「フッ化物」 **resistant**「抵抗力のある」 **decay**「虫歯」 **oral**「口の」 **expanded**「拡張した」 **administer**「～をおこなう」 **place**「～をおく」 **anesthetics**「麻酔薬」 **restoration**「修復」

Exercise 6 : LISTENING （テープを聞いて，空所を埋めなさい。）

1. (   ) (   ) that he has done his homework.

2. He (   ) foreigners (   ) an enterprise.

3. The (   ) (   ) smoking and cancer is close.

7. Amino Acids （未来の予防薬，アミノ酸）

　We now know that many of the amino acids not only serve as structural components of proteins, but also serve as factors in various crucial biochemical functions, just as the vitamins and minerals do. And, beyond vitamin and mineral-type functions, the amino acids are also critical to the function of the brain.

　We also know that though several amino acids can be made by the body it doesn't necessarily mean that the body is making enough for all its needs. Evidence suggests that various factors may prevent the body from synthesizing enough amino acids. In some cases, diseases or stresses of all kinds combine with genetic and metabolic factors to cause amino acid deficiencies. In years to come, amino acids may equal vitamins and minerals as therapeutic agents in sickness, and preventive agents in health.

serve as「～として役に立つ」　**crucial**「大変重要な」　**biochemical**「生化学上の」　**critical**「重大な」　**not necessarily**「必ずしも～でない」　**synthesize**「合成する」　**combine with～to...**「～と結びついてその結果…する」　**genetic**「遺伝学上の」　**deficiencies**「欠乏，不足」　**in years to come**「来るべき数年後に」　**therapeutic**「治療上の」　**agents**「薬剤」

Exercise 7 : WRITING　（本文中の語句を参考にして，次の日本文を英文になおしなさい。）

1. 確かに彼は勤勉家だが，堅物というわけではない。

2. 風邪のため東京ドームでの巨人・阪神のナイターを観戦できなかった。

3. 来る21世紀は不確実性の時代になると言われている。

8. The Pros and Cons of Abortion （人工中絶の賛否）

 The arguments for and against abortion are widely known. The moral objection is based primarily on the contention that human life begins with the union of the egg and the sperm, so that destruction of the fertilized ovum is an act of homicide. Opponents of abortion hold that it opens the door to the brutalization of society, encouraging "mercy deaths," infanticide, and other violation of the sanctity of life.

 The defenders of abortion take the position that the embryo does not become a human being until after a certain time, fixed variously from 12 to 28 weeks of gestation. Their arguments for abortion are based on the premise that the overriding consideration should be the health of the prospective mother and child.

pros and cons「賛否両論」 **egg**＝egg cell. **fertilized ovum**「受精した卵子」 **mercy death**「安楽死」 **infanticide**「嬰児殺し」 **sanctity of life**「生命の尊厳」 **embryo**「胎児」 **gestation**「懐妊期間」 **premise**「前提」 **overriding**「優先的な，支配的な」 **prospective mother**「近く母親になる女性」

Exercise 8 : LISTENING　（テープを聞いて空所を埋め，和訳しなさい。）

1. Techniques for abortion are (　　　　) in some of the oldest medical texts (　　　) to man.

2. The (　　　　) of abortion goes back to human tradition far older than the earliest (　　　) history.

3. In ancient Greece, Plato (　　　　) abortion to limit the size of the population and (　　　) an economically healthy society.

9. The Effect of Laughter （笑いの効用）

At the school of Medicine of the University of California, Los Angeles, doctors have been trying to find out if emotions affect the chemistry of the human body. As the result of recent research, they have found out that specific changes take place throughout the body as the result of human attitudes.

Every emotion, negative or positive, makes its registrations on the body's system. When you are ill, you had better read every humorous book you can get. The goal is to be uplifted and relieved of worry and panic through laughter.

Laughter is a form of internal jogging. It moves the organs around. It enhances respiration. It is an igniter of great expectations.

take place＝happen「おきる」 **uplifted**「精神的に元気が出る」 **be relieved of**「～から解放される」 **internal**「体の内部の」 **enhance**「増す」 **respiration**「呼吸」 **igniter**「火つけ役」

Exercise 9 : WRITING （与えられた書き出しを用いて，英訳しなさい。）

1. 来週ジュネーブで平和会談がひらかれる。
   The Peace Talks...

2. 子供たちが無事だときいてほっとした。
   I was...

3. 教師として彼は学生たちに学習意欲をたきつける能力をもっている。
   As a teacher, he...

10. How to Enjoy Drinking （酒の上手なのみ方）

Alcohol abuse is a serious problem. But if we understand there is a safe way to drink, alcohol can do more good than harm.

First, the manner of drinking is important. One should always sip slowly. As 20％ of alcohol is absorbed directly from the stomach into the bloodstream, gulping alcohol produces a sudden, marked rise in the alcohol level in the blood and hence in the brain.

Secondly, we should eat something while drinking, preferably protein or fatty products. Food covers the stomach wall, sponges up the alcohol and carries it gradually through the digestive process, slowing absorption and allowing the metabolism and brain to adapt.

alcohol abuse「アルコール中毒」 **do good**「益がある」（↔ do harm） **sip**「すする」 **absorb**「吸収する」 **blood stream**「血管」 **gulp**「ガブのみする」 **marked**「著しい」 **fat**「脂肪」 **preferably**「好ましくは」 **digestive**「消化の」 **metabolism**「代謝作用」 **adapt**「適応する」

Exercise 10: WRITING （日本語のヒントをもとに，英文を完成しなさい。）

1. This medicine will （3語）_____.
   [あなたに効くでしょう]

2. （2語）_____ can truly affect a way of
   [食事の作法]
   life of British people.

3. The extra money will （7語）_____.
   [新しい車を買うのを可能にしてくれる]

11. How to Promote Health （健康増進のために）

A balanced diet, or balanced physical activity, to promote health is easy neither to define nor measure. People who eat one type of food to excess may make up for that disadvantage in some other respect. And manual workers who are spectators rather than active sportsmen include those who have to exert physical strength and agility in their everyday jobs.

Again, the data can be interpreted in other ways than in relation to level of knowledge or education, or personal responsibility. Commercial advertisements are planned to 'educate' tastes, and the education provided in schools is not always calculated to prepare young people to ward off influences upon their consumption and behaviour which may be undesirable for health.

to excess「過度に」 **make up for**「～を埋め合わせする」 **disadvantage**「不利な条件」 **respect**「点」 **spectator**「観客」 **exert**「～をつかう」 **agility**「敏捷性」 **the data** （スペースの関係で統計図表を省略）イギリスでは高収入者は糖分摂取量が比較的少なく，専門職の者は労働者より喫煙量が少ない。また，年齢により好みのスポーツも異なり，50,60代はゴルフ，30,40代はテニス，10,20代 はスカッシュ等々の資料。
in relation to「～に関して」 **not always**「必ずしも～でない」 **be calculated**「考えられている」 **ward off**「～を避ける」 **consumption**「消費」

Exercise 11: WRITING　（カッコ内の語(句)を用いて，英訳しなさい。）

---

1. あらゆる点で彼女は正しい。（respect）

2. 彼はスピードをあげて遅れを取り戻した。（make up for）

3. 健康によくない行動は避けなさい。（ward off）

12. Vocational Rehabilitation Counselor （社会復帰カウンセラー）

Vocational rehabilitation counselors use work as a method of assisting the physically or mentally disabled to develop and live to their full potential. Through interviews and special tests, counselors assess clients' skills and abilities to develop vocational goals that will help them achieve maximum independence and functioning.

During the counseling process these professionals advise their clients about job opportunities and training availability, and assist them in training and job placement. They also provide counseling to help clients adjust successfully to a new work situation. Counselors work with a variety of patients ranging from those who have never worked at all and who may be considered unemployable, to those returning to work.

vocational「職業としての」 **disabled**＝handicapped. **potential**「可能性」 **assess**「～を判断する」 **maximum**「最大の」 **functioning**「役目」 **availability**「有効性」 **assist**「～を助ける」 **placement**「職業紹介」 **adjust to**「～に適応する」 **range from ... to**「…から～にいたる」 **those**＝those who.

Exercise 12 : LISTENING （テープを聞いて，空所を埋めなさい。）

1. The contents of an index (　　　) (　　　) A to Z.

2. It is not easy for me to (　　　) (　　) new situations.

3. (　　) (　　　) (　　) patients came to the counselors.

13.　Almighty Germanium　（万能のゲルマニウム）

　Believe it or not, one of the most exciting and promising supplements is a rare mineral used in making transistors! The Japanese who have always had a knack for finding new ways to use transistors, have done most of the research on this nutrient. And they have found that it can 1) improve mental alertness, 2) lower high blood pressure, 3) act as a potent anti-inflammatory, 4) raise endorphin levels by inhibiting the enzyme that destroys these natural analgesics, 5) rapidly stimulate interferon production to fight infections, especially viruses, 6) suppress tumors in animal experiments, 7) boost the immune system.

　Germanium is not stored in the body, so 100 percent of what is taken in is excreted within two or three days. Thus there is no toxicity from excess storage, as there can be with other minerals. To date, the only nontoxic form of this mineral is the sesqui-oxide form.

knack「こつ」　**mental alertness**「精神的敏捷性」　**potent**「強力な」　**anti-inflammatory**「抗炎症剤」　**endorphin**「エンドルフィン；脳や下垂体に存在し，ストレス等の侵害要因で血中に分泌する物質」　**enzyme**「酵素」　**analgesics**「鎮痛剤」　**interferon**「インターフェロン；ウイルス増殖抑制物質」　**infections**「感染症」　**tumors**「腫よう」　**boost**「増大する」　**excrete**「排泄する」　**toxicity**「有毒性」　**storage**「貯蔵」　**to date**「今までのところ」　**sesqui-oxide**「三二酸化物」

Exercise 13: WRITING　（本文中の語句を参考にして，次の日本文を英文になおしなさい。）

1. 嘘だと思うだろうが，ゲルマニウムは高血圧にきくそうだ。

2. 現在までのところ，これ以上の情報は判明していません。

3. 彼は観光客に同時通訳のアルバイトをしています。

14. Calcium and Adult Diseases （カルシュウムと成人病）

Calcium has only recently been identified as a nutrient that can help prevent cancer, especially colorectal cancer. In this form of cancer, the normal balance between abnormal cell growth and normal growth in the bowel shifts to favor abnormal growth. Calcium can actually reduce abnormal cell growth in the bowel and restore equilibrium to the extent that the bowels of high-risk people more closely resemble those of low-risk people.

Calcium is also a factor in preventing cardiovascular disease by lowering blood pressure. Several recent studies have pointed out that low levels of calcium in the diet can lead to high blood pressure, and high calcium levels seem to offer some protection. In one study, calcium supplements were effective in lowering blood pressure in women with high blood pressure, whereas it had no effect in women with normal blood pressure.

colorectal「結腸・直腸の」 **bowel**「腸」 **abnormal**「異常な，病的な」 **favor**「～を助長する」 **equilibrium**「平衡状態」 **to the extent that**「～の程度まで」 **cardiovascular**「心臓・血管の」 **point out**「指摘する」 **lead to**「～に至る」

Exercise 14 : LISTENING （テープを聞いて空所を埋め，和訳しなさい。）

1. When it comes to (　　　) prevent degenerative disease, chromium is the (　　　) that really shines.

2. One of the (　　　) that we have so much cardiovascular disease is the high level of (　　　) in our diet.

3. Too much insulin is secreted to (　　　) with all the sugar, and the excess insulin is believed to damage the blood (　　　).

15. Dr. Waksman, Father of Antibiotics
（抗生物質の父，ワクスマン博士）

　In contrast to the discovery of penicillin by Fleming which was largely due to a matter of chance, the isolation of streptomycin was the result of long-term, systematic research by a large group of workers. The initiator and leader of this group was Dr. Waksman. He had been actively engaged on research work on soil microbes, and concluded that the disappearance of the tubercle bacilli in the soil was due to the influence of other antagonistic microbes.

　It was Dr. Waksman who introduced the new word "antibiotic," and it represents an antibacterial substance, produced by a microbe which is antagonistic in action to another.

Dr. Waksman(1888-1973)ロシア生れの米国の細菌学者。Nobel 医学生理学賞(1952)
antibiotic「抗生物質」　**long-term**「長期間の」　**isolation**「分離」　**microbe**「微生物」
tubercle bacilli「結核菌」　**antagonistic**「拮抗する」

Exercise 15 : WRITING　（与えられた書き出しを用いて，英訳しなさい。）

1.　ストレプトマイシンのおかげで，以前は致命的な病いであった結核を制圧することができるだろう。
　　Thanks to streptomycin, ...

2.　我々はついに結核への最初の効果的な治療薬を手に入れた。
　　At last, we have got ...

3.　新しい治療薬の発見にはいつも長期的な研究が必要である。
　　Long-term research ...

16. The Insulin Factory （インシュリン工場）

Every cell in the human body is a chemical plant. Among the many products manufactured for export are hormones: messenger proteins that carry instructions from their site of production by way of the bloodstream to other cells throughout the body, where they regulate a variety of functions. One hormone is insulin, whose primary role is to control the transport of glucose, the body's main energy source, from the bloodstream into the cells where it is burned.

An insulin deficiency impairs the body's ability to get glucose into the cells. As a result glucose accumulates in the blood, leading to the condition known as diabetes. Uncontrolled, diabetes can severely reduce life expectancy.

site「場所」 **impair**「損なう」 **blood stream**「血流」 **deficiency**「不足」 **diabetes**「糖尿病」 **life expectancy**「寿命」

Exercise 16 : WRITING （日本語のヒントをもとに，英文を完成しなさい。）

1. Hormones are called messenger proteins because they carry instructions

   _____
   （6語）
   ［体中の他の細胞に］

2. （5語）_____ is (to) control the transport
   ［インシュリンの主な役割は］
   of glucose.

3. （6語）_____, people
   ［もしグルコースが血中にたまると］
   will have diabetes.

17. Unconscious Dying Patients （生命維持の是非）

Although she was not dead by the applicable medical criteria for determining brain death, the medical authorities were satisfied that there was no hope that she would ever recover to a cognitive state : she was characterized as being in a 'chronic, persistent, vegetative condition,' kept alive only with the assistance of the respirator.

In those circumstances, the parents of Karen Quinlan decided that it would be best for her to be removed from the life-support machine. Accordingly, her father applied to the court to be appointed her guardian and claimed that, as guardian, he would be entitled to authorize the discontinuance of all 'extraordinary' medical procedures sustaining Karen Quinlan's vital processes and hence her life.

The Supreme Court of New Jersey upheld the father's claim.

applicable「適切な」 **criteria**「基準」 **cognitive**「認識力のある」 **chronic**「長期にわたる」 **vegitative condition**「植物人間状態」 **respirator**「人工呼吸装置」 **life-support**「生命維持の」 **accordingly**「そこで」 **guardian**「後見人」 **be entitled to**「～の資格がある」 **authorize**「～を認定する」 **sustain**「～を持続させる」 **vital**「生命に関る」 **Supreme Court**「州最高裁判所」 **uphold**「～を支持する」

Exercise 17 : WRITING （カッコ内の語(句)を用いて，英訳しなさい。）

1. 彼は年金を受ける資格がある。(be entitled to)

2. 彼が生きている見込みはない。(There is no hope)

3. 我々は自国の伝統を絶やさないでおくべきである。(keep ～ alive)

18. What Are Interferons ? （インターフェロンとは）

　Interferons are proteins that exert a wide-spectrum antiviral activity in animal cells and also possess several biological activities other than the ability to induce an antiviral state. An interferon is often active only in cells of the animal species producing that interferon; cellular metabolic processes involving both RNA and protein synthesis are required for development of interferon activity. Concentrations of interferons that induce significant levels of biological activity usually cause little or no toxic effect on cells. Interferon production is induced by viruses or a number of antiviral substances.

　Interferons were discovered in the late 1950s by Isaacs and Lindenmann, who were working then at Mill Hill in London.

protein「蛋白質」 **exert**「行使する」 **wide-spectrum**「広範囲の」 **antiviral**「抗ウイルス性の」 **induce**「誘導する」 **cellular**「細胞状の」 **metabolic**「新陳代謝の」 **RNA**「リボ核酸」 **synthesis**「合成」 **concentration**「凝縮したもの」 **substance**「物質」 **interferon**「ウイルス抑制因子」ウイルスの感染に応じて生じ，その成長を阻む働きをする蛋白質。

Exercise 18 : LISTENING　（テープを聞いて，空所を埋めなさい。）

1. In many ways, (　　　) are ideal antiviral substances.

2. Only recently has some progress been made in finding (　　　　) antiviral drugs.

3. Viruses or a number of antiviral substances induce interferon (　　　).

19.　Allergies　（アレルギー体質）

　A decade ago, to most people the word "allergy" meant hay fever, or respiratory distress caused by particles of dust, pollen, or hair floating in the air. Few people were aware that the concept of allergy was being extended to the very food we eat.

　Being allergic to something means your immune system has become sensitized so that it identifies that substance or thing as not self and, in effect, declares war on it every time you come in contact with it. The immune system has a very efficient memory so that it never forgets an invader with whom it's done battle. This is a remarkable ability, one that saves our lives many times over.

　But in many people this immune memory also causes allergies. The immune system is primed by genetic factors or sensitized early in life to recognize a normally harmless substance such as pollen or fur as a danger, and reacts with an immune show of force that can leave you feeling miserable.

hay fever「花粉症」　**respiratory distress**「呼吸困難」　**pollen**「花粉」　**sensitized**「敏感になって」　**self**「同質物」　**in effect**「実際に」　**every time**＝whenever.　**come in contact with**「～に触れる」　**invader**「病原体」　**many times over**「何度も繰り返して」　**is primed**「予め教え込まれて」　**genetic factors**「遺伝学的要因」

Exercise 19：WRITING　　（本文中の語句を参考にして、次の日本文を英文になおしなさい。）

1.　アレルギー反応は免疫組織が原因と言われる。

2.　春は花粉のため，一年中で一番やっかいな季節です。

3.　僕は子供の頃から，にんじんが大嫌いだ。

20. How to Lose Weight on a Diet （ダイエットによる減量）

About two-thirds of the adults in the U. S. are either on a diet or believe they should be. Dieting to lose weight is a way of life for most Americans.

We assume, first of all, that the principal goal of a diet is to lose weight. Achieving that goal is not difficult, theoretically. It's the magic of actually making it happen—and making it stay happened—that is full of mystery. A lot of things get in the way. And every new diet that's invented promises to remove those obstacles in a new way. To make your diet more effective and lasting, we will recommend supplements that can help you:

1. Increase the efficiency of digestion／2. Promote the metabolism of fat, carbohydrates, and protein／3. Stimulate energy／4. Reduce cravings／5. Suppress the appetite and calm the nerves.

nutrients「栄養剤」 **theoretically**「理論的に」 **supplements**「ビタミン，ミネラル等の補給剤」 **get in the way**＝obstacle. **carbohydrates**「炭水化物」 **protein**「蛋白質」 **cravings**「強い欲求」

Exercise 20 : LISTENING　（テープを聞いて空所を埋め，和訳しなさい。）

1. Most people take it for (　　　) that the body is just going to burn (　) for fuel whenever it needs to.

2. If you increase the efficiency of your (　　　　) while on a diet, you will (　　) more nutrients and be more satisfied.

3. When we don't get all the nutrients we need, the body's deep (　　　) for better nutrition is (　　　　) in our own desire for more food.

21. The Mind-Body Effect （心と身体の関係）

An increasing number of scientists now contend that the body's healing system and its belief system are closely related. That is why hope, faith, and the will to live can be vital factors in the war against disease. One crucial factor that influences the system of belief and healing is the attitude of the physician. One of a doctor's main functions is to engage to the fullest the patient's own ability to mobilize the forces of mind and body in turning back disease. The patient's belief in the judgment and healing power of the physician is often more important than the treatment itself. Dr. Herbert Benson, an associate professor of medicine at Harvard Medical School, believes that a doctor's "caring" about his or her patient causes specific physiological improvement.

contend＝maintain「主張する」 **healing system**「病気を治し、健康になろうとする働き」 **belief system**「信念による働きかけ」 **vital**＝crucial「非常に重要な」 **to the fullest**「できるだけ十分に」 **turn back**「進行をくいとめる」 **"caring"**「心くばりのある世話」

Exercise 21 : WRITING （与えられた書き出しを用いて、英訳しなさい。）

1. 身心の相関関係を重視する医師が増えている。
   An increasing number of ...

2. そういうわけで病院には希望にみちた、力強い雰囲気が大切である。
   That is why ...

3. 強い意志をもつ患者ほど病気の進行をくいとめるのに成功する傾向がある。
   Patients with a strong will ...

22. Treatment of Child's High Fever
(子供の高熱の手当て)

Between the ages of 1 and 5 years, children may develop fever as high as 104° at the onset of mild infections, such as colds, sore throats, grippe. On the other hand, a dangerous illness may never have a temperature higher than 101°. So don't be influenced too much by the height of the fever. And it is well to remember that the fever is not the disease. The fever is one of the methods the body uses to help overcome the infection. It is also a help in keeping track of how the illness is progressing.

In one case the doctor wants to bring the fever down because it is interfering with the child's sleep or exhausting the patient. In another case the doctor is quite willing to leave the fever alone, and concentrates on curing the infection.

onset「発病」 **infection**「感染」 **grippe**＝influenza. **keep track of**「～の跡を追う」 **interfere with**「～のさまたげになる」 **exhaust**「疲労させる」 104°F＝40°C. 101°F＝38.3°C.

Exercise 22 : WRITING　（日本語のヒントをもとに，英文を完成しなさい。）

---

1. He was badly exhausted (5語) _____
　　　　　　　　　　　　　　　[熱の出はじめに]

2. (5語) _____ that each person
　　[～だとおぼえておいた方がよい]
　has great potential abilities.

3. The sound of TV upstairs (4語) _____ .
　　　　　　　　　　　　　　　　[私の仕事のさまたげになった]

23. Mental Health （心の健康）

In the past no one could understand mental illness. Magic charms were used to drive away 'evil spirits.' Until the days of Philippe Pinel patients were treated cruelly.

In recent years doctors have made some interesting discoveries. For example, they have discovered that when a certain part of the brain is injured the patient loses his power of speech. And when the left side of the brain is damaged the muscles of the right side of the body are affected. They have found the exact parts of the brain which control important actions of the body. Surgeons now take a special interest in the brain and the nervous system.

An American, Harvey Cushing, learned how to take tumours from the brain. These growths press against delicate parts of the brain and cause mental disturbances.

charm「お守り」 **drive away**「追い払う」 **evil spirits**「悪霊」 **take(an)interest in**「～に興味をもつ」 **affect**「～を冒す」 **growth**「腫瘍」 **cause**「～を引き起こす」 **disturbances**「不安」 **Philippe Pinel** (1745-1826) フランスの精神病の治療, 看護法の改革者。 **Harvey Cushing** (1869-1939) アメリカの外科医。

Exercise 23 : WRITING （カッコ内の語(句)を用いて，英訳しなさい。）

1. 災難よけのお守りがしばしば使用されてきた。(charm)

2. トムはとくに歴史に興味がある。(interest)

3. 私はうるさい蝿を外へ追い払った。(drive)

24. Prevention of Influenza （インフルエンザの予防）

The mainstay of prevention is the use of inactivated influenza virus vaccines. These vaccines provide about 80 per cent protective efficacy. The antigenic composition is reviewed annually so that the vaccine contains the most recently circulating strains. Usually the vaccine is a trivalent product containing one or more subtypes of influenza A and B.

The recent vaccines have been purified by density gradient centrifugation or chromatography and have very low reaction rates. One or two per cent of persons vaccinated will have fever and systemic symptoms peaking at 8 to 12 hours after vaccination and up to 25 per cent may have mild local reactions at the site of vaccination.

mainstay「ささえる主要な者」 **inactivated**「不活性化した」 **efficacy**「効力」 **antigenic**「抗原の」 **composition**「合成物」 **annually**「毎年」 **circulating strains**「普及している種類」 **trivalent**「3価の」 **subtype**「亜類型, 特殊型」 **density**「濃度」 **gradient**「だんだんあがる」 **centrifugation**「遠心分離」 **chromatography**「色層分析」 **systemic**「全身の」 **symptoms**「症状」 **mild**「軽い」 **at the site of**「〜のところに」

Exercise 24 : LISTENING （テープを聞いて，空所を埋めなさい。）

1. The air has (   ) (   ) by the aircleaner.

2. You have the (   ) (   ) your father's car, don't you?

3. I hope you won't catch (   ) (   ), because (   ) is contagious.

25. A War against AIDS （エイズとの戦い）

It's a dangerous world, there's no question about it. And it doesn't seem to be getting any less dangerous, either. The entire medical world has been mobilizing for a war against one of the most insidious and deadly disease ever known—AIDS, or, Acquired Immune Deficiency Syndrome.

While scientists wrestle with the research and try to come up with a new medical miracle to combat this dread disease, most of us watch the ever-escalating statistics and wonder what we can do to protect ourselves and our beloved ones. At this point, we can do two things:

1. Hope and pray that the research will yield some answers and some effective drugs as soon as possible.
2. Apply what we know about the prevention of other viral diseases and general support of the immune system to our personal health programs.

AIDS「後天性免疫不全症候群」 **mobilizing for**「～のため動員される」 **insidious**「潜行性の」 **deadly**「致命的な」 **wrestle with**「～に全力を尽くす」 **come up with**「～を供給する」 **viral**「ウイルス性の」 **immune system**「免疫組織」

Exercise 25: WRITING （本文中の語句を参考にして,次の日本文を英文になおしなさい。）

1. 彼はエイズの原因研究に取り組んでいる。

2. 医学界全体が死に到る病,エイズ撲滅のための新薬開発に努力している。

3. 君はできるだけ速く定期検診を受けるべきである。

26. Diet and Cancer （食事と癌）

Sometimes you not only need to add nutrients to your diet to improve your health and prevent cancer, but you also need to remove some things. To lessen your risk of breast cancer, you should also decrease the amount of fats and oils in your diet. Several studies bear out the fact that as fats in the diet rise, so does the risk of breast and colon cancer.

It's unfortunate that for the past 20 years we have been oversold on the value of polyunsaturated vegetable oils. Although use of these oils may result in lower cholesterol levels than the use of saturated oils or animal fats, they can also result in higher levels of free radicals in the body. The free radicals, in turn, can raise the risk not only of cancer, but also of heart disease.

colon「結腸」 **fats**「脂肪質」 **oils**「油性物」 **bear out**「立証する」 **oversold**「吹聴され過ぎて」 **polyunsaturated**「多不飽和の」 **saturated**「飽和した」 **free radicals**「遊離基」 **in turn**「今度は，逆に」 **intake**「摂取」

Exercise 26 : LISTENING　（テープを聞いて空所を埋め，和訳しなさい。）

1. Vitamin A has always been known to (　　　) the immune system, but we know that beta-carotene (　) immune function independently.

2. Studies have shown that women with diets (　　　) in beta-carotene and vitamin C have less (　　) of developing cervical cancer.

3. So (　　　) is the effect of beta-carotene that it can (　　　) reverse as well as prevent the abnormal growth of cervical cells.

27. The Nature of AIDS （エイズの性質）

  As recently as a decade ago, it was widely believed that infectious disease was no longer much of a threat in the developed world. The remaining challenges to public health there, it was thought, stemmed from non infectious diseases and degenerative diseases. This confidence was shattered in the early 1980's by the advent of AIDS. In spite of the startling nature of the epidemic, science responded quickly.

  In the two years from 1982 to 1984 the outlines of the epidemic were clarified, a new virus — the human immuno-deficiency virus(HIV)—was shown to cause the disease, a blood test was formulated and the virus's targets in the body was established.

infectious「伝染性の」 **the developed world**「先進諸国」 **stem from**「～からおこる」 **degenerative**「細胞の変性による」 **shatter**「うちくだく」 **immuno-deficiency**「免疫不全」

Exercise 27 : WRITING　（与えられた書き出しを用いて，英訳しなさい。）

1.　日本人は教育に関心の高い国民であると広く信じられている。
　　It is widely believed that ...

2.　AIDS の到来により世界は新たな困難に直面しなければならなかった。
　　With the advent of AIDS, the world ...

3.　伝染のおそれにもめげずダイアナ妃はエイズ患者と握手をしてはげました。
　　In spite of the fear of transmission, Princess Diana ...

28. German Measles （風疹）

The rash of German measles looks much like the rash of real measles, but the two diseases are entirely separate. In German measles there are no cold symptoms (running nose or cough). There may be a little sore throat. The fever is usually low. A doctor should make the diagnosis, because German measles is easily confused with real measles, scarlet fever, and certain virus infections.

It is bad for a woman to have German measles during the first three months of pregnancy because of the chance of her baby acquiring defects from the disease. German measles vaccine should be given to all children, particularly girls, between the ages of 1 year and puberty.

German measles「風疹」（別名 Rubella） **rash**「発疹」 **real measles**「はしか」 **running nose**「鼻水」 **sore throat**「のどのいたみ」 **scarlet fever**「猩紅熱」 **puberty**「思春期」

Exercise 28 : WRITING　（日本語のヒントをもとに，英文を完成しなさい。）

---

1. (3語) _____ he's going to have an ear infection.
   [～しそうである]

2. I'm always _____ ruby _____ garnet.
   [とりちがえる]

3. There are some kinds of (2語) _____.
   [経口ワクチン接種]

[33]

29. What Should an A. I. D. Child Be Told?
(精子提供者の匿名義務)

　The Law Commission's proposal to deem an A. I. D. child born to a married couple to be the child of that couple would continue and strengthen the trend towards concealment of A. I. D. origin. The Warnock Committee too recommends that the donor retains his personal anonymity. Two major reasons support this trend. First, the apparent father will very likely not wish his infertility to be known even to the child.

　The object of A. I. D. is to give a couple a child as near to their own as possible. Second, donors may well be unwilling to come forward if many years after they donated sperm they face the prospect of being confronted by their 'children' and consequent possible disruption of the families they may by then have founded.

A. I. D. = artificial insemination by donor「夫以外の男子の精子による人工受精」 **deem** = think. **concealment**「隠匿」 **donor**「精子提供者」 **anonymity**「匿名」 **infertility**「生殖力のないこと」 **as 〜 as possible**「できるだけ〜」 **unwilling**「いやがる」 **confront**「直面する」 **consequent**「結果として起こる」 **disruption**「分裂」

Exercise 29: WRITING　（カッコ内の語(句)を用いて，英訳しなさい。）

1. 彼は舞踏会に行く気持ちになれなかった。(unwilling)

2. 出来るだけ早くきてほしいのですが。(possible)

3. その時までに彼らは，家庭の分裂に直面するかもしれない。(then)

30. Factors of High Blood Pressure
（高血圧の諸原因）

Psychosocial factors. The role of psychosocial factors in the pathogenesis of hypertension has aroused considerable interest. There is little evidence that harm can result from short-term blood pressure increases in response to acute psychological stimuli. On the other hand, there are reports that factory workers subjected continually to intensive noise have higher mean blood pressures than others working in quieter surroundings in the same factory. Studies on migrant populations indicate that long-term exposure to adverse psychosocial circumstances might lead to hypertension.

Alcohol. An association between a high intake of ethyl alcohol and high blood pressure has been reported in a number of studies, but the mechanism of the association remains unclear.

psychosocial「社会的，心理的」 **pathogenesis**「発病」 **hypertension**＝high blood pressure. **short-term**「短期の」 **stimuli**(*pl*)「刺激」 **migrant**「移住してきた」 **subject ... to**「…を～にさらす」 **adverse**「逆境の」 **association**「関連」

Exercise 30 : LISTENING　（テープを聞いて，空所を埋めなさい。）

1. Sickness often (　　　) (　　　　) eating too much.

2. The patient suffering from skin cancer was (　　　　) (　　　) X-rays.

3. His performance (　　　　) (　　　　) (　　　　　) of the audience.

31. A Godsend for Ulcers （潰瘍の天与の妙薬）

This may seem like a joke, but to thousands of people suffering from ulcers, the information that cabbage juice can heal ulcers has been a godsend. It's also a fascinating story of how circumstances can combine to make a treatment that is on the brink of revolutionizing standard medical care for disease and turn it into one of the most well-kept secrets on earth.

First, the secret: Raw cabbage juice, administered two or three times a day, can relieve pain from ulcers and immediately and drastically reduce the time required for healing. This treatment was researched, developed, and tested by Dr. Garnett Cheney in the 1940s. His work began with animals and culminated in controlled, double-blind experiments in which the effects of cabbage juice were tested against the effects of a placebo. His results were consistent. Cabbage juice always reduced pain and sped up the healing process.

ulcer「潰瘍」 **godsend**「思いがけない幸運」 **combine to**「結びつき～になる」 **on the brink of**「～の寸前である」 **well-kept**「良く守られた」 **administered**「処方された」 **drastically**「徹底的に」 **developed**「開発されて」 **culminate in**「～で絶頂に達する」 **double-blind**「二重盲検の」 **placebo**「偽薬」

Exercise 31: WRITING （本文中の話句を参考にして，次の日本文を英文になおしなさい。）

1. 天気も良く，グループの気も合ったので，ピクニックは成功だった。

2. 彼らは食料が切れて餓死寸前だった。

3. クリスマス・パーティは最高潮に達してプレゼントが配られた。

32. How to Thrive on Stress （ストレスを逆用する）

Real life is impossible without stress. There is no way to completely avoid it. Yes, some ways of life are less stressful than others, but total deprivation from stress is impossible. If you somehow manage to isolate yourself completely from stress, that isolation itself will be stressful.

Besides, we like stress. We have an appetite for it, and if it's not appeased, we starve. Stress is wear and tear, but without it, there can be no growth and repair. We need a certain amount of stress to stimulate body and mind.

Unfortunately, life in the modern world brings with it stresses we can live without, such as anxiety and pollution of our air, water, and food supplies.

Stress upsets our balance. All living things try their best to achieve and maintain balance. Not only do whole organisms try to maintain balance, but individual systems within organisms.

deprivation「解放」 **manage to**「どうにか～する」 **isolate yourself**「～から隔離する」 **wear and tear**「消耗すること」 **repair**「良好な整備状態」 **live without**「～なしで生きる」 **try their best**「最善を尽くす」 **organisms**「有機的生活体」

Exercise 32 : LISTENING （テープを聞いて空所を埋め，和訳しなさい。）

1. When we're ticking along and the body is in (　　　　　), all our biological (　　　) operate in harmony.
2. Stress (　　　　　) us by upsetting our balance and using up our (　　　) to restore balance.
3. Stress puts (　　　　　) on all our biological machinery that works to maintain the balance in our (　　　).

33. Heart Transplant （心臓移植）

　When Dr. Christian Barnard began performing some of the world's first heart transplants in 1967, such efforts usually ended in failure and death because the patient's immune system rejected the implanted heart. But the development in 1980 of the antirejection drug cyclosporin has brought a big change.

　Now more than 200 heart transplants are being performed in the U.S.A., and the survival rate is about 80％ for a year, 50％ for five years (statistics in 1984).

　Recently, an operation of artificial-heart implant took place in the U.S.A. Like a landing on the moon, it was an event that aroused a sense of awe at the incredible powers of technology, a sense that almost anything that can be imagined can be done.

Christian Barnard (1922-　) 南アフリカ共和国の心臓外科医。　**immune system**「免疫機構」　**reject**「拒絶する」　**implant**「埋めこむ」　**antirejection drug cyclosporin**「拒否反応抑制剤シクロスポリン」　**artificial-heart**「人工心臓」

Exercise 33 : WRITING　（与えられた書き出しを用いて，英訳しなさい。）

---

1. もし重い心臓病にかかっているとしたら，心臓移植の手術を受けたいと思いますか。
   Suppose you had ...

2. そうですね，それは手術の成功率によります。
   Well, it would depend on ...

3. 最近のハイテク医療の進歩は全くめざましいですね。
   Recent progress of ...

34. Cell Division ; Initiator of Life's Fire （生命の火を燃やすもの）

A skinned knee heals. A cancerous tumor grows. An embryo develops into a baby. Underlying all these commonplace events is one of the most extraordinary natural phenomena known to science—the ability of one living cell to transform itself into two living cells.

Cell division is the act that has kept life's fire burning for billions of years, relaying its spark from old cell to new.

In every tissue, there are regulatory mechanisms that tell a cell when to divide and when not to divide. Failures in these mechanisms lead to some of the most catastrophic diseases and birth defects.

initiator「反応を起こさせるもの」 **skin**「皮をむく」 **tissue**「組織」 **tumor**「腫瘍」 **embryo**「胎児」 **catastrophic**「悲劇的な」 **relay**「中継する」 **birth defect**「生まれつきの欠陥」

Exercise 34 : WRITING （日本語のヒントをもとに，英文を完成しなさい。）

1. Since World War II, Japan ____(4語)_____
   […へと変化してきた]
   an advanced industrial power.

2. Please tell me ____(3語)_____ this experiment.
   [いつ始めたらいいか]

3. Egoism ____(2語)_____ isolation.
   [〜へと通じる]

35. The Black Death （黒死病）

In the fourteenth century the streets in the towns and cities were very narrow. Black rats were everywhere searching for food. They were found in the dirty streets and in the houses. Their bodies were covered with the fleas which caused the plague.

The Black Death was an infectious disease. This means that it passed quickly from one person to another. It spread quickly, like a fire. It was passed on in the breath. It was so infectious that people thought they could catch it from someone who only looked at them.

People who had the plague were not allowed to leave their homes. Their families, too, were kept indoors. Red crosses were painted on the doors. The crosses warned everyone of the danger. Sometimes wooden boards were nailed across the door.

plague「ペスト」 **the Black Death**「黒死病（ペスト）」14世紀ヨーロッパに大流行し人口の4分の1をも死滅させた疫病。 **in the breath**「あっというまに」 **infectious**「伝染性の」 *cf*. contagious「接触伝染性の」 **be allowed**「～が許される」 **warn ... of**「…に～について警告する」 **nail**「～に釘付けする」

Exercise 35 : WRITING　（カッコ内の語(句)を用いて，英訳しなさい。）

1. 教授会では禁煙になっています。(be allowed)

2. 彼女はうんといったかと思うとすぐいやという。(in the same breath)

3. テレビニュースは台風の接近を警告した。(warn ～ of)

36. Four Humors （4つの体液の意味）

Galen regarded the production and excretion of the *yellow* bile and of the more toxic black bile as the functions of both liver and spleen. These humors, especially when present in abnormal quantities, were regarded as the cause of various diseases. The third humor, the *phlegm* was considered as a composite matter. Phlegm, a collective expression for a number of body fluids, was made responsible for a multitude of ailments, especially dropsy and ascites.

Health, he thought, was based on the balance of the unmodified four principal humors, their 'symmetry,' an idea which antedates Hippocrates and was first clearly expressed by Alcmaeon in Sicily.

the four humors 4体液説は古代ギリシャ時代の病気の原因は4種の体液，粘液（Phlegm），黄胆汁（yellow bile），黒胆汁（black bile），血液（blood, 快活）の量的バランスが乱れることにあるとしたことに因る。　**Galen** [géilin]（130？-200？）「ガレヌス」古代医学を集大成した。　**excretion**「排出」　**yellow bile**「黄胆汁，=choler, かんしゃく」　**toxic**「毒性の」　**black bile**「黒胆汁，=melancholy, 憂鬱」　**spleen**「脾臓」　**composite**「合成の」　**phlegm**「粘液，冷静」　**dropsy**「水腫」　**ascites**「腹水症」　**Hippocrates** [hipǽkrətiːz]（460？-355？）「ヒポクラテス」，医学と父の呼ばれるギリシャ医学の最高峰。

Exercise 36: LISTENING　（テープを聞いて，空所を埋めなさい。）

1. (　　　)(　　　) carries the quality of melancholy.

2. (　　　) carries the quality of coolness.

3. (　　　)(　　　) carries the quality of choler.

37. The Hospice Movement （ホスピス運動）

　Hospice is part of a movement to humanize the way medical care is given. This movement has focused on the beginning as well as the end of life. Natural childbirth and the hospice movement both share the common recognition that the family has an important role to play in the health care system. The family understands needs that are beyond the knowledge of the health professional. The family and patient working in concert with the doctor and the nurse can form the most compassionate plan of care.

　The family is the basis and the strength of our society. Our families are strengthened by sharing and participating in the death of a loved one. Our lives revolve around our loved ones. Why should life just before death be any different?

　Hospice is a reality and a bright light in our health care system. Hospice provides a type of care that must become a model not just for the dying but for the whole health delivery system.

focus on「～に焦点を合わせる」 **beyond the knowledge of**「～の知らない」 **in concert with**「～と協調して」 **compassionate**「真心のこもった」 **not just ... but**＝not only ... but also. **delivery**「分娩，出産」

Exercise 37 : WRITING　（本文中の語句を参考にして,次の日本文を英文になおしなさい。)

1. 我々はホスピス運動に多大な関心を寄せるべきである。

2. 彼らは日本がもっとアジアの国々に目を向けるべきという共通の認識をもっている。

3. 日本は今世界経済において重要な役割を負っている。

38. How We Get Old （老化の仕組）

The aging clock is used to explain all the causes of aging that we do not yet understand. After all the random and accidental causes of aging are examined, there still seems to be a limiting factor somehow built into the body, which ages us. Some theories hold that the aging clock is within the cell, and that the cells of the body can reproduce only a limited number of times. Some theories state that the aging clock exists in the DNA molecule, which purposely transmits faulty information once we have lived enough time to bear offspring and pass on our genes. Other theories state that the aging clock is in the brain or endocrine system, and that a "death hormone" is secreted, which stimulates all of the age-related deteriorations in structure and function.

DNA=deoxyribonucleic acid「デオキシリボ核酸」 *cf*. RNA. **molecule**「分子」 **offspring**「子孫」 **genes**「遺伝因子」 **endocrine system**「内分泌組織」 **secreted**「分泌する」

Exercise 38 : LISTENING　（テープを聞いて空所を埋め，和訳しなさい。）

1. Today we know that thinking, imagination, and other brain functions are (　　　) or discouraged by the brain's biochemical (　　　　).

2. Moreover, we know that (　　　) "in your head" can also influence many (　　　) of your physical condition.

3. We do not recommend drastically cutting caloric (　　　) unless the diet is carefully (　　) to provide a density of nutrients and proteins.

[43]

39. Plasticity in Brain Development （脳の発達）

Even though the basic organization of the brain does not change after birth, details of its structure and function remain plastic for some time, particularly in the cerebral cortex. Experience—sights, smells, tastes, sounds, touch and posture—activates and, with time, reinforces specific neural pathways while others fall into disuse. The developing brain can be linked to a highway system that evolves with use: less traveled roads may be abandoned, popular roads broadened and new ones added if needed.

plasticity < **plastic**「可塑的・可変的」 **cerebral cortex**「大脳皮質」 **neural**「神経の」 **be linked to** = be compared to. **reinforce**「強化する」 **evolve**「徐々に発展する」

Exercise 39 : WRITING （与えられた書き出しを用いて，英訳しなさい。）

1. 脳のある部分は生後も可塑的であり続けることがわかっている。
    Some parts of the brain …

2. 経験が特定の神経回路を発達させる。
    Experience develops …

3. この話からすると脳は使うことによって次第に発達するようだ。
    This sounds like …

40. How and Why Do We Dream? (夢の不思議)

20th-century psychologists, psychiatrists, and doctors have come up with some interesting facts about dreams. Everybody dreams every night. Everybody dreams in color; if awakened in the middle of a dream, you will report it in brilliant technicolor, but if awakened 15-plus minutes after a dream, you may remember a dream but in black and white. And dream-deprived people become irritable, anxious, less tolerant in stressful situations.

We may have dreams because we have needs that are unmet in our daily lives. Freud used dreams in an attempt to solve people's psychological troubles.

Dreams can be a vehicle for knowledge not open to the waking mind.

psychiatrist「精神分析医」 **come up with**「提示する」 **deprive**「奪う」 **irritable**「怒りやすい」 **tolerant**「寛容な」 **vehicle**「媒介物，表現手段」 **Freud, Sigmund** (1856-1939) オーストリアの医師，精神分析学の開祖。主著『夢判断』(1900) 他。

Exercise 40: WRITING （日本語のヒントをもとに，英文を完成しなさい。）

1. A team of psychiatrists _____(6語)_____
   [新しい解決法を示した]
   _____ for the patients with severe mental corruption.

2. New scientific discoveries should _____(5語)_____.
   [いかなる国に対してもひらかれている]

3. We owe much to Freud, who is the _____(3語)_____.
   [精神分析学の始祖]

41. The Beveridge Plan （福祉国家をめざして）

There is the idea of making pensions not a birthday present to be got when you become 65, but pensions to be given on retirement and increasing as retirement is postponed. Then there are the family allowances. That, I think, is the greatest of all the revolutions in this scheme. There is far better provision for housewives and widows. There is the abolition of the approved society system, on which I shall have a word to say later.

Finally, there is the death grant. Honourable Members may wonder whether the introduction of the death grant is really a major change. I suggest that it is, having regard to the history of this proposal.

pension「年金」 **family allowances**「家族手当て」 **provision**「備え」 **abolition**「廃止」 **approved society**「認可組合」 **introduction**「導入」 **grant**「補助金」 **Honourable Members**「英国下院議員」 **regard**「敬意」 **William Beveridge** (1879-1963) イギリスの経済学者，社会学者。「完全雇用，社会保障計画」で有名。

Exercise 41 : WRITING　（カッコ内の語句を用いて，英訳しなさい。）

1.　彼は慶応大学の入学試験に来年うかるかしら。(whether)

2.　自動化の導入は当時は革新的であった。(introduction)

3.　彼女は将来，看護婦になろうと思っている。(an idea of)

42. Liability of Nursing Staff （看護の意味）

Nurses, as well as doctors, may sometimes make mistakes. All that has been said in relation to doctors applies equally to them. A nurse will be judged in accordance with the standard of skill and carefulness to be expected of a nurse in this position and speciality with this seniority. A midwife must show a midwife's skill. It is not enough, for example, to display only the standard of an S. R. N. who has done 13 weeks obstetrics. The midwife holds herself out as a specialist.

There are a few decided cases relating to nurses. A nurse who either failed to notice or act on evidence of a lump in a patient's breast when she examined her at a Family Planning Clinic was held to be negligent. She should have taken steps to ensure that the patient's incipient cancer was properly investigated.

apply to「～に適用される」 **in accordance with**「～に合わせて」 **seniority**「在職年数優先」 **midwife**「助産婦」 **S. R. N.**＝state-registerd nurse. **obstetrics**「産科学」 **hold oneself out**「～と主張する」 **case**「訴訟例」 **negligent**「怠慢な」 **ensure**「～を確実にする」 **incipient**「初期の」 **properly**「適切に」

Exercise 42：LISTENING （テープを聞いて，空所を埋めなさい。）

1. You (　　　) (　　　) (　　　) steps to avoid troubles.

2. He (　　　) (　　　) (　　　) as a distinguished scholar.

3. As might be (　　　) (　　　) a gentleman, he was as good as his word.

\multicolumn{3}{l}{A SHORTER COURSE IN GOOD HEALTH}

A SHORTER COURSE IN GOOD HEALTH
5分間健康・医療・看護   [B-213]

| 1 | 刷 | 2004年4月5日 |
| 8 | 刷 | 2021年4月1日 |

著　者	瀬谷幸男　　Yukio Seya
	西村月満　　Tsukimaro Nishimura
	中山　潤　　Jun Nakayama

発行者	南雲　一範　Kazunori Nagumo
発行所	株式会社　南雲堂
	〒162-0801　東京都新宿区山吹町361
	NAN'UN-DO Publishing Co., Ltd.
	361 Yamabuki-cho, Shinjuku-ku, Tokyo 162-0801, Japan
	振替口座：00160-0-46863
	TEL: 03-3268-2311（代表）／FAX: 03-3269-2486

製版所	壮光舎印刷
装　丁	銀月堂+nagilaz
検　印	省　略
コード	ISBN4-523-17213-7　C0082

Printed in Japan

E-mail　nanundo@post.email.ne.jp
URL　http://www.nanun-do.co.jp/